QUICK POUNDS SHED

HOW TO GET FAST WEIGHT LOSS AND FITNESS WITHOUT EXTREME HUNGER

AVA WELLSPRING

DESCRIPTION

Want to lose weight fast and safely without starving or sweating? This book will show you how to do it with a 30-day meal plan based on your body type and metabolism. You will also learn the science behind weight loss and the benefits of healthy eating. Order Quick Pounds Shed today and get ready to transform your body and life!

TABLE OF CONTENT

Copyright © 2023 Ava Wellspring...................... 2

DESCRIPTION.. 3

TABLE OF CONTENT...................................... 4

CHAPTER ONE.. 5

Getting Started.. 5

The Quest For Fast Weight Loss...................... 8

The Relationship of Fitness And Extreme
Hunger.. 9

CHAPTER TWO..15

Discovering Your Body Type............................15

The Science of Weight Loss............................. 16

The Function of Metabolism............................24

Your Body Chemistry....................................... 27

Regular Diet... 32

CHAPTER THREE.. 39

Crafting out a useable Timeline...................... 39

Determining Your Ideal Weight...................... 47

Setting Realistic Goals......................................50

CHAPTER FOUR... 53

Tips for Meal Planning..................................... 53

Creating a Balanced Diet plan for 30 days....... 78

List of 30 meals to consider............................. 83

The Importance of Nutritious Rich Foods....... 90

Benefits of Healthy Eating for Adults.............. 95

Benefits of Healthy Eating for Children.......... 96

CONCLUSION.. 97

CHAPTER ONE

Getting Started

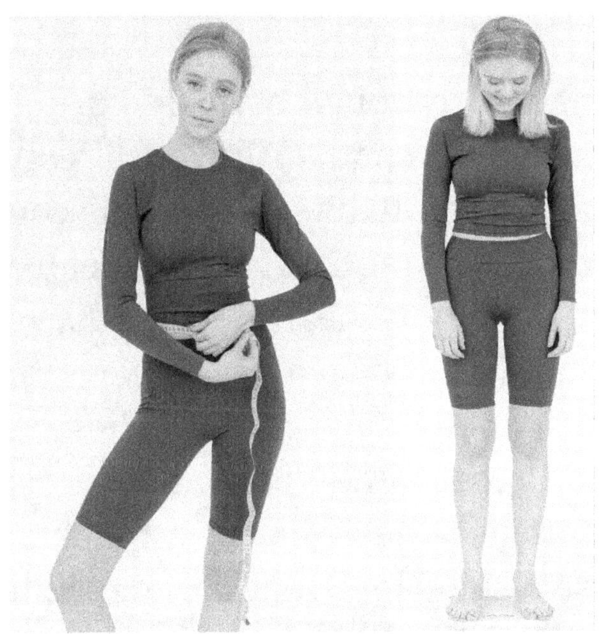

Ensure to keep track of a fast metabolism diet that requires eating different types of foods in different aspects to boost your metabolism and burn fat. This diet allows you to consume a lot of carbs and fruits, proteins and vegetables, and healthy fats and oils at designated phases. This phase could be within 30 days and repeated till it becomes a lifestyle.

Make sure you are ready to make permanent changes in your lifestyle and health habits. Try to discover your inner motivation, set realistic goals, enjoy healthier foods, get proactive, stay hydrated always, and learn to manage stress. These are the most effective and proven strategies that will aid a quick and fast weight loss that do not require counting calories or following a must-to-follow diet

Another thing to note is to reduce your hunger by eating more protein, fiber, and healthy fats. These nutrients can make you feel fuller for a much longer time and reduce your ergonomic appetite. You can also drink water before meals, eat mindfully, and avoid distractions while eating. Consciously practice habits that can help you eat less without feeling deprived

Lose substantial weight without diet or exercise by making some simple changes in your daily routine. For example, you can choose to chew your food slowly, consume smaller plates of food, resting effectively, avoiding sugary drinks, and moderately eating spicy foods. These tips can help you reduce your calorie intake and boost your metabolism naturally

The Quest For Fast Weight Loss

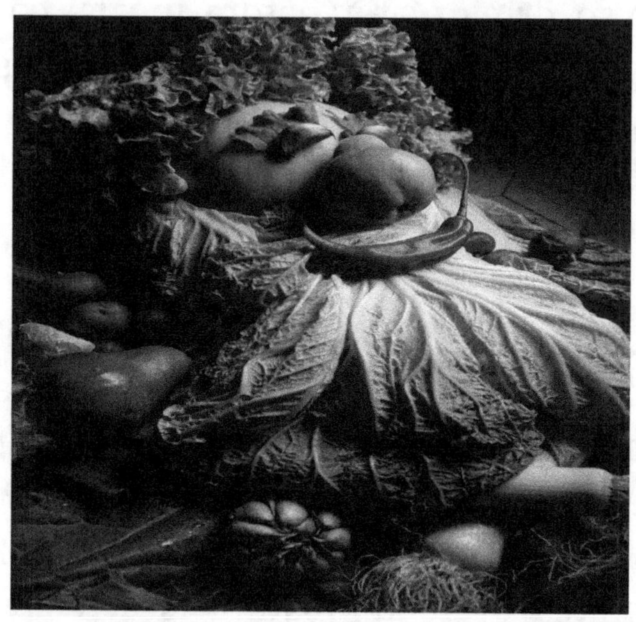

The relative search for a quick loss in weight is quite a common one, but it can also be quite alarming and less effective. There are several methods and diets online that claims to help you lose weight very fast, but they may not be based on scientific evidence or suitable for your individual needs. Why? This is because we have different body types which is also based on our body chemistry.

The Relationship of Fitness And Extreme Hunger

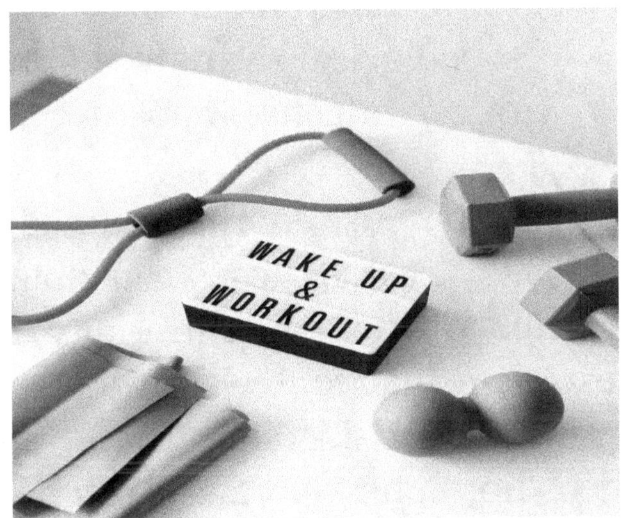

The relatedness of physical fitness and hunger is diverse and it involves many core factors, such as the following:
- Categories
- Magnitudes
- Exercise duration

- The external characteristics, hormonal harmony and the level of competence with fitness of the individual's body and;
- The environmental and psychological variables that greatly influences appetite.

In relation to enormous study, vigorous exercise can contribute greatly to the concentrations of hormones that controls satiety and optimum satisfaction. There are such hormones produced by the body which are ghrelin and leptin that contributes substantially to appetite levels. Fat cells produces leptin and this leptin notifies the brain to reduce hunger substantially when energy intake is sufficient. Ghrelin is produced by the stomach and small intestine and springs up hunger when the stomach is empty. Exercise can decrease ghrelin levels and increase leptin levels, which can lead to reduced appetite levels.

These effects however, may likely vary based on the type of exercises undertaken. Most studies suggest that rigorous exercises, such quality exercises done at intervals can suppress appetite much more than regular exercises like walking and jogging. This could be because enormous and painstaking exercises triggers a stress response that inhibits signs of hunger and unsatisfaction. On the contrary, usual and moderate exercises may skyrocket the appetite levels so much by triggering the consumption of energy which may leads to the deficit in calories.

The body's composition of fats and endurance level is a major factor to consider which could influence the way exercise affects hunger. Som evidence indicates that obese individuals have In Obesed individuals, the lower levels of leptin sensitivity, meaning that their brains do not respond to leptin signals as effectively as lean individuals. This may result in a continuous feeling of severe hunger even after exercise. On the contrary, the lean and strong ones may end up with higher levels of leptin sensitivity and experience greater appetite degradation after a vigorous exercise.

Finally, the environmental and psychological factors could have great influence on the way exercise affects hunger. For instance, different people might have studied associations between body exercise and the consumption of food, such as helping themselves out with a good treat after a tedious day job or just by eating much more which is their way of rewarding themselves for calories. Many others might be influenced by external influences, for example the smell or sight of food, their inner emotions, or media practices. These other factors has the power to override the physiological push for hunger and satiety and could result in people to eating less or much more than they need.

Informatively, fitness and extreme hunger are closely related concepts that relies on core influences and other external factors. Performing exercise consistently can have a whole different feel on hunger which relies on the different types, vigorousity, and the duration with the time intervals for the different exercises. The body composition of the person, competence level, hormonal harmony, and the psychological and environmental influences that impact appetite is also a key consideration of how much or quick exercise will impact the feel of hunger. So, it is very necessary to pay attention to your body's response to hunger and satiety and to eat a wholesome balanced diet that meets the requirements of your nutritional and physical fitness needs.

CHAPTER TWO

Discovering Your Body Type

Finding out your body type can assist you in knowing better while understanding your physique and tailoring your fitness and nutrition plans in the proper way. Generally, there are three well-known body types which are:

1. **The Ectomorphs**: They usually happen to be lean and do face a challenging period accumulating weight or muscle. They usually have a very quick metabolism and could find it really difficult to get through muscle accumulation.

2. **The Mesomorphs**: They usually tend to portray more physical and muscular build. They tend to amass

weight and rapidly lose fat quite easily, which makes them very suitable for different kinds of physical fitness activities that involves physical contact.

3. The Endomorphs: They generally do have a greater percentage of body fat and usually find it much easier to accumulate a lot of weight, which includes body fats and muscle. This is often because they have a much slower nutrient metabolism.

The Science of Weight Loss

The quantity of calories an individual consumes and sheds must have some alterations so the person can lose right amounts of fats in order to lose weight or regulate body weight. The body which has a calorie deficit or loses more calories than absorbed will likely lose more weight than a body that accumulates more calories. With this started, the scenario really seems understandable, balanced and straightforward but so many factors necessary to be considered cues up our calorie intake and output.

According to Dr. Kindel, he discovered that there are a range of procedures that regulate food intake via our brain impulses and auxiliary organs that makes available to us, signs for feelings surrounding satiety and hunger. Our body does control the amounts of food burned or the level of energy consumption, and it performs this by addressing our metabolic rate and processes, which are usually impacted by the body hormones, ailments, and medicines.

The study of weight loss is so complicated than just maintaining records of calories consumed and spent. The key is not just losing weight but also maintaining a sound and healthy modification to your diet based on your body type, such as maximizing the quality and quantity of whole fruits and vegetables while limiting and discouraging yourself from the intake of beverages with added sugar, trans fats and other sugary foods.

Losing weight is a very sturdy scientific approach that is affected by several things. The various important elements to note are:

1. Calorie balance: The necessity for a balance between the calories you consume from the intake of food and drinks and the calories you dissipate through physical exercise and metabolism serves as the key to weight reduction. Most times, you must constantly be able to used up more calories than the calories you consume which causes calorie deficit, so that reduction in weight will be easily achievable.

2. Metabolic rate: Several influential factors like age, genetics, gender, and amounts of muscle all have a great influence on our metabolic rate. Basal metabolic rate is referred to as the quantity of

calories your body requires, in order to accomplish vital bodily processes . Your Basal metabolic rate could surge-up by simply building muscle mass through high-end exercises and resistance training.

3. Diet: What matters in diet consumption is the quantity and quality of the food absorbed. Weight loss could be greatly appreciated by a very quality choice of diet that contains rich proteins, carbohydrate complexes, advantageous fats, and lots of fruits and veggies. It is also important to pay attention to the proportions.

4. Doing exercises. Workouts could really aid calorie dissipation and storage of muscular mass. Cardiovascular exercises and core exercises that aids muscle build-up (such as jogging or cycling) can inclusively help you in reducing weight.

5. Weight reduction is impacted by core things to consider which includes stress, sleep quality, and hormonal balance. For instance, inadequate rest and continuous subject to stress might result in weight gain.

6. Cognitive attitude: Weight Loss is majorly affected by lifestyle and attitudes. It is very necessary to avoiding

eating in ignorance. It is also mindful of one to create achievable goals and objectives, and strive to adopt right culinary eating habits and avoid emotional snacking always.

7. Hydrolysis: The Intake of water is necessary for the optimum health of the body and it is most times a misleading concept for the feel of hunger and appetite.

8. Medical Conditions: illnesses of several kinds, including polycystic ovarian syndrome and thyroid dysfunction, can create serious impact on the overall body weight. It is important to consult a doctor or a healthcare expert If you

are suspecting a hidden issue with your health.

9. Genetics: Your overall body natural weight with how it responds to food and physical activities could be affected or counted by genetics. Your choice of lifestyle, despite the huge role genetics play, could still have a significant impact on weight

10. Consistency: In order to maintain the right weight for a healthy body system, it is necessary to consider making long term modifications to your diet and exercise pattern. Rapid weight loss and strong approaches to losing weight are good but could become useless for the long term if

drastic measures are not applied to your lifestyle.

It is necessary that you approach weight loss from the perspective of being an effective and efficient way of maintaining good body shape. Interacting with a certified dietician or a professional in health could save you some good time and aid you in getting unique personal advice directed towards crucial need and unique goals.

The Function of Metabolism

The chemical procedures and reactions that occur in living organisms to permit and protect life is referred to as metabolism. Three core purposes of metabolism co-exist:

- To convert food energy into cellular energy which the body cells can make use of, for different bodily functions, which includes body movements, tissue repairs, and additionally, external and internal growth of the tissues and organs.

- To change food nutrients into the fundamental elements need by living organisms, such nutrients include lipids, protein, nucleic acids (DNA), with some sugars and carbohydrates.

- To completely eliminate metabolic byproducts produced by metabolic processes such as water, urea and carbon-dioxide.

The distinct known types of metabolic procedures / processes are Anabolism and catabolism. The building process of storing energy and producing new organic molecules is known as anabolism. The catalytic breakdown of molecules made up of organic matter plus energy which results into wasted products and energy is known as Catabolism. Substances like enzymes and hormones could serve as catalysts to quicken the reactions. These substances also help in regulation of these two processes.

Several factors such as environmental conditions, gender, age, muscle mass, diet and physical activity, have an impact on metabolic processes. The metabolism of an individual, which obtains the quantity of calories the person burned and how much of body weight gained or lost, is usually different from person to person. In addition, some people have a hard time maintaining their energy balance or metabolising distinct substances like medicine due to metabolic issues in the person's system. For example , a metabolic condition, diabetes in particular, really have negative effects on how the body absorbs carbohydrates and glucose.

Your Body Chemistry

Based on various grounds, there is a dire need for a much deeper awareness of your body chemistry/composition. Knowing this, can aid you in gaining greater insights and appreciating how your body works, how it engages with the surrounding environment, and the way it reacts to a number of stressors. Acknowledging this could indeed help you in making well informed decisions with regards to your medical condition, diet, nutrition, and lifestyle.

Your total body composition is composed of several chemical constituents, scientific compounds, and interactions that usually occur in your cells, tissues, organs, and systems. The core fundamentals that makes up your body chemistry are:

- The chemical constituents which makes up your body: There are about 60 chemical constituents that have been discovered in the body, but what their core functions are, is yet to be discovered. There is approximately 96 percent of the total mass of the human body that is made up of just four basic elements which are oxygen, carbon, hydrogen and nitrogen, with so much of it in the physical appearance of water. The other 4% represents a small sample amount of elements in the periodic table .

- The smaller particles that comprise your body: The human body entails several kinds of molecules that does a lot of critical work. The most notable ones include proteins, lipids, carbohydrates, nucleic acids, and water. Proteins which serve as enzymes, antibodies, hormones and locomotors are also the core building components of your body cells and tissues. Lipids, which include fats and oils that preserve energy, safeguard your body, and build up cell membranes. Starches and different forms of complex and simple sugars are considered as carbohydrates that nourishes the body with energy and structural support. Nucleic acids are DNA and RNA which both store, retain and carry genetic information. Body molecules are absorbed and conveyed by a solvent known as water.

- The rules and regulations that guide your life: All through our lives chemical processes perpetually take place in our body which gives us the strong ability you need to grow, move around, think, reproduce and make concrete decisions. These collective fundamental processes are known as metabolism, which is subdivided into two types: anabolism and catabolism. Anabolism is the accumulation process of retaining energy while building up or producing new organic materials. Catabolism is the breakdown process of disi°ntegrating energy and organic materials resulting in waste products and energy. These two activities are regulated by the hormones and enzymes, which serves as mediators to accelerate the reactions.

- The coherence that preserves your health: For the best results, your body's composition needs to be retained in a homeostatic or balanced condition. This actually translates that a range of specified factors, including temperature, pH, blood pressure, blood sugar, oxygen level, etc., needs to be taken care of. Numerous illnesses or medical conditions could develop if these factors deviate too far from the normal range. Your body uses a variety of feedback loops using sensors, controllers, and effectors to monitor and adjust these parameters.

Regular Diet

Numerous chemicals in a typical diet, some of which contain trace elements, are being studied for their effects. We can only be certain of about 20 elements' actions at this time. Here is a brief summary, with brackets denoting the percentage of body weight.

The majority of the body's weight, or roughly 60%, is made up of water, which also contains the majority of oxygen (65%) and hydrogen (10%). Life would be virtually impossible without water.

Life (18%) and carbon go hand in hand. It plays a crucial role because it possesses four bonding sites that enable the construction of lengthy, intricate chains of molecules. Furthermore, the dynamic organic chemistry that occurs in our cells is made possible by the fact that carbon bonds may be generated and broken with only a small amount of energy.

The amino acids that make up proteins and the nucleic acids that make up DNA all include three percent nitrogen.

The most prevalent mineral in the human body is calcium (1.5%), which is almost entirely found in bones and teeth. Ironically, calcium plays a crucial part in several biological processes like protein regulation and muscular contraction. In reality, if a person's diet is deficient in calcium, the body will actually remove calcium from bones, which can result in issues like osteoporosis.

Phosphorus (1%) is primarily found in bone but is also present in the molecule ATP, which gives cells the energy to power chemical reactions.

An essential electrolyte (one that carries a charge in solution) is potassium (0.25%). It is essential for nerve electrical signalling and for regulating the heartbeat.

Two essential amino acids that play a key role in giving proteins their form contain sulphur (0.25%).

Another electrolyte that is essential for electrical signalling in nerves is sodium (0.15%). Additionally, it controls the body's water balance.

The negative ion chloride, which contains 0.15 percent of chlorine, is typically found in the body. This electrolyte is crucial for preserving a healthy fluid balance.

Magnesium (0.05%) is a mineral that is crucial to the skeleton and muscle structure. More than 300 crucial metabolic reactions also require it.

A crucial component in the metabolism of practically all living things is iron (0.006%). Haemoglobin, the substance that carries oxygen in red blood cells, also contains it. The majority of women don't consume enough iron daily.

0.0037 percent of fluorine is found in bones and teeth. It does not seem to be important to physical health outside of preventing tooth decay.

All forms of life require the trace metal zinc (0.0032%). The "zinc fingers" found in a number of proteins help control genes. Dwarfism has been linked to zinc deficiency in underdeveloped nations.

Copper (0.0001%) plays a crucial role as an electron donor in a number of biological processes.

Copper is necessary for iron to function effectively in the body.

Making thyroid hormones, which control metabolic rate and other cellular activities, requires iodine (0.000016%). Iodine deficiency is a significant health issue that affects a large portion of the world's population and can cause brain damage and goitre.

For some enzymes, including numerous antioxidants, selenium (0.000019%) is necessary. There are numerous reports of selenium poisoning from consuming plants cultivated in selenium-rich soils, despite the fact that plants do not appear to need selenium for living like animals do, although they do absorb it.

By interacting with insulin, chromium (0.0000024%) helps control blood sugar levels, albeit the precise mechanism is yet unclear.

You can decide which chemicals are required for the body to function effectively by understanding body chemistry. Nutritionists use this method to decide which foods are ideal for preserving health. For instance, vitamins are a crucial group of chemicals that support bodily processes like the development of healthy bones, the production of blood cells, and the efficient operation of your metabolism. You can determine what foods to eat to receive these vitamins by knowing what vitamins are required for each of these processes.

CHAPTER THREE

Crafting out a useable Timeline

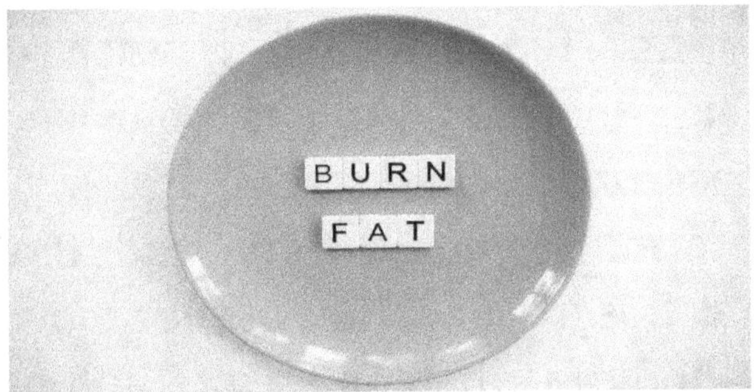

For countless people, losing weight is an everyday objective, but it may also be difficult and discouraging. There is no one-size-fits-all strategy for losing weight because a variety of factors can influence how quickly and successfully you can do it. However, creating a personalised and realistic timeframe will assist you in organising your weight reduction quest and maintaining motivation.

You can use the methods below to create a practical timeline for weight loss:

To start, figure down how much you weigh now as well as your body mass index known as BMI). To determine your weight and BMI, which is a calculation of the amount of body fat that takes into account your height and weight, you will require a scale and a BMI calculator, accordingly. A BMI of 18.5 pounds to 24.9 pounds is considered healthy, while a BMI of 25 pounds or more suggests overweight or obesity.

2. Define a sensible target for weight loss. You can anticipate to lose approximately 4−8 pounds (1.8−3.6 kg) each month at a secure and durable rate of weight reduction of 1-2 pounds (0.45−0.9 kg) per week.

However, your beginning weight, age, sex, and degree of activity may change this. Based on your present weight, height, age, sex, and level of activity, a weight loss calculator can help you determine how long it will take you to reach your target. Alternatively, you could decide to lose 5–10% of your body weight in the next six months.

3. Pick a dietary strategy that complements your interests and way of life. Finding a diet that you can follow for the long run is more crucial than choosing one of the many different diets that promise to help you lose weight. You may acquire the nutrients and energy you need to lose weight healthily by eating a balanced diet that includes a range of foods from all food groups, such as fruits, vegetables,

whole grains, lean proteins, healthy fats, and dairy products. To keep track of your calorie intake and usage, you can also utilise a calorie tracking app or website.

4. Add some exercise to your regular regimen. You can avoid weight regain, increase muscle mass, burn calories, and enhance your mood by exercising. It is generally advised to engage in strength training exercises at least twice per week in addition to 150 minutes of moderate-intensity aerobic activity or 75 minutes of vigorous-intensity cardiovascular activity per week. Additionally, you can raise your non-exercise activity thermogenesis, which is the amount of energy you expend performing regular tasks like cleaning, gardening, and walking.

5. Monitor your development and modify your strategy as necessary. You can track your progress using a variety of techniques, including regular self-weighing, body measurements, body fat analysis, and self-portrait photography. However, little variations or plateaus are expected and common during the weight loss process, so don't let them deter you. Instead, concentrate on the progress you have made and recognise your accomplishments. If you see that your weight loss has slowed down or stopped altogether for longer than a few weeks, you may need to adjust your diet or exercise programme to break through the plateau.

Here is an illustration of how to create a useful timescale using this approach:

- Actual weight: 90.7 kg (200 lbs)
- Obese at 30.9 BMI at now.
- Target weight reduction of 160 pounds (72.6 kg)

One pound (0.45 kg) of weight is lost each week with an estimated 40 weeks to attain the objective.

Dietary pattern: Mediterranean diet and Physical activity: thirty minutes per day of vigorous walking and 20 minutes per week of strengthening exercises

Progress monitoring: Weekly weight check and monthly waistline measurement

Timeline: Week 1: Begin eating a Mediterranean-style diet and exercising for thirty minutes each day.

Week 2: Add strength training activities three times each week.

Week 4: Assess yourself and keep track of your body weight.

Week 8: Measure yourself and keep track of your bodyweight. Also, measure your waist and keep track of it.

Week 12: Document your weight by weighing yourself.

Evaluate yourself and note your weight in Weeks 16 and 20. In Week 16 you should also measure your waist and record that information.

- Week 24: Gauge yourself and note it, as well as measuring your hips and thighs and noting it.

- Week 28: Note your weight by weighing yourself.

- Week 32: Measure your waist circumference and weight, and keep a record of both.

- Week 36: Document your weight by weighing yourself.

- Week 40: Gauge yourself, note it, determine your hips and thighs circumference, comparing it to your initial measures, and acknowledge your success.

As you progress through, you may always change your plan. Enjoying the adventure and being pleased with yourself for achieving healthy changes to your physical and mental health are the most crucial things.

Determining Your Ideal Weight

Your optimum weight can be determined in a variety of ways based on how tall you are, gender, age, and type of body. Utilising the body mass index (BMI), which is a proportion of your weight to height, is among the most used approaches. For both men and women, a healthy BMI range is between 18.5 and 24.9 pounds. However, BMI does not take into account elements that may have an impact on your weight, such as muscle mass, distribution of calories, ethnic background or medical issues. Because of this, it is not a flawless indicator of your wellbeing or looks.

Utilizing algorithms that determine your perfect body weight depending on your height and gender is an additional strategy. These equations were initially created for medical applications, such as calculating medicine dosages, but they are now also applied in several sports to categorize athletes by weight classes. The Robinson, Miller, Devine, and Hamwi mathematical equations are only a few of the well-known formulas. These equations do have some drawbacks, though, as they frequently overestimate or undervalue the appropriate weight for certain heights. Additionally, they do not take into account personal preferences, variances in bone form, or body shapes.

A more modern technique is to calculate your optimum weight using an equation that includes your height and BMI. A 2016 study that revealed this equation to be highly correlated with the BMIs of 22.5 for men and 21 for women—which are roughly in the centre of the optimal BMI range—led to its development. The calculation looks like this:

Height measurements in inches less 60 is equal to 5 x BMI + (BMI divided by 5) x Body Weight in pounds.

Height measured in metres less 1.5 divided by (2.2 x BMI + 3.5 x BMI) yields weight in kilogrammes.

If you are taller or shorter than normal, this equation may give a more precise estimate of your optimal weight than the earlier ones.

Setting Realistic Goals

Your ability to set reasonable objectives and set achievable targets can help you succeed in several spheres of life, including social, academic, professional, and personal ones. Here are various justifications for, instructions on how to do so, and occasions to do so:

Why: By establishing attainable objectives and targets, you can:
   - Establish a distinct direction and goal for your efforts
   - Encourage yourself to act and overcome obstacles
   -Enhance your efficiency and effectiveness while monitoring your

accomplishments and outcomes. Promote your sense of self–worth and trust.

How: Establishing attainable objectives and targets entails:

- Outlining your goals and objectives in a precisely achievable, specific, quantifiable, relevant, and time–bound method;

- assessing your resources, advantages, disadvantages, setbacks, possibilities, and dangers that could deter you from achieving your goals;

- determining your time frame for completing the goals and objectives.

- Based on input and evolving conditions, reevaluate and modify your aims and objectives as necessary.

- Integrating your goals and objectives into your everyday routine and future plans.

- Assessing your successes, rejoicing in them, and taking lessons from your setbacks.

When: You can establish objectives and goals at any time, but they are particularly helpful when you:

- Begin an entirely novel venture, task, or endeavor;

- Address an issue or obstacle that needs a remedy or improvement;

- Desire to learn new abilities or cultivate an existing one;

- Want to adjust an existing routine or behavior that has held you back;

- Are interested in going after something you love or enjoy that makes you happy.

CHAPTER FOUR

Tips for Meal Planning

These are quick and easy ways to make meal planning a successful habit.

1. Begin modestly

It could seem a little overwhelming if you've never made a meal plan or if you're just starting out again after a long break.

Making a beneficial change in your life, such as developing a habit of meal planning, is the same. It's a good idea to start modest and gradually gain confidence to make sure your new habit is enduring.

Just a few meals or snacks for the coming week should be planned at first. You'll eventually learn which planning techniques are most effective, and then you may gradually expand your strategy by including other meals as you see fit.

2. Think about every food group

Whether you're planning meals for a week, a month, or just a few days, it's crucial to include foods from each food category.

A well-rounded diet prioritises whole foods such as veggies, fruits, whole grains, legumes, high-quality protein, and healthy fats while lowering sources of processed grains, artificial sugars, and too much salt.

Consider each of these food groups as you browse through your favourite recipes. Make it a point to fill in the blanks if any of them are missing.

3. Establish order.

Any good meal plan must have a strong foundation in organisation.

Since you'll be aware of exactly what you have on hand and where your equipment and materials are, having an organised kitchen, pantry, and refrigerator makes everything from creating menus to grocery shopping and meal preparation a breeze.

Your meal prep areas can be organised in any way you choose.

Make sure it's a system that functions for you, though.

4. Spend money on high-quality storage bins.

One of the most important tools for meal preparation is food storage.

Meal preparation may be particularly difficult if you're currently dealing with a pantry full of mismatched containers with missing lids. Putting money and time into premium containers is a wise decision.

Think about the intended usage of each container before making a purchase. Make sure you select containers that are safe for freezing, microwaving, or dishwasher cleaning if you intend to do any of those things with the food.

Glass containers are microwave-safe and environmentally friendly. They are widely accessible both offline and online.

Additionally, having a range of sizes for various food types is useful.

5. Maintain a fully stocked pantry.

An excellent method to speed up meal preparation and make creating menus easier is to keep a foundation stock of pantry essentials.

Foods that are nutritious and flexible to keep in your pantry:

Brown rice, quinoa, oats, polenta, bulgur, and other healthy grains

Legumes: pinto beans, lentils, garbanzo beans, and dry or canned black beans

Foodstuffs that can be canned include tomatoes, tomato sauce, artichokes, olives, corn, fruit without added sugar, salmon, tuna and poultry.

Olive, avocado, and coconut oils

Baking necessities: flour, cornflour, baking soda, and baking powder

Others include peanut butter, potatoes, mixed nuts, dried fruit, and almond butter.
When you stock up on some of these fundamental necessities, you only

need to worry about buying fresh things when you go grocery shopping once a week. This can help you feel less stressed and make meal planning more effective.

6. Always have an array of spices on hand

A meal's amazingness or lacklusterness can be determined by the herbs and spices used. A meal plan that routinely includes delectable foods may be sufficient for the majority of people to develop the habit of meal planning.

Herbs and spices are excellent flavour enhancers in addition to being rich in plant components that have a number of health advantages, including less cellular damage and inflammation.

Pick and purchase a couple of jars of your favorite dried herbs and spices each time you go grocery shopping if you don't already have a sizable supply.

7. First, look in your pantry.

Take stock of what you already have on hand before sitting down to prepare your meals.

Look through your pantry, freezer, and refrigerator as well as the rest of your food storage spaces and make a list of any particular things you wish to use up or that you need to.

By doing this, you may use up the food you currently have, cut down on waste, and avoid making unnecessary purchases of the same products.

8. Always show there on time

Making meal preparation a priority is the greatest way to incorporate it into your daily life. Regularly setting aside a period of time only for planning can be beneficial.

Making a food plan can take as little as 10-15 minutes each week for some people. You could need a few hours if your plan calls for portioning meals and snacks or pre-preparing specific food products.

Making time and maintaining consistency are essential for success, regardless of your particular method.

9. Establish a location for storing and preserving recipes.

By keeping them in a place where you can easily access them whenever you need to, you can save the unneeded frustration of attempting to recall recipes.

This could be in a physical space in your home or in a digital format on your computer, tablet, or smartphone.

Meal planning can be less stressful and time-consuming if you keep a place set out for your recipes.

10. Request aid

It can be difficult to consistently stay motivated to create a fresh menu every week, but you don't have to go it alone.

Do not be reluctant to consult your family members if you are in charge of organising and preparing meals for a large household.

If you cook mostly for yourself, ask your pals what they're making or get ideas from online sources like social media or food blogs.

11. Compile a list of your favorite foods.

Forgetting a dish that you or your family truly enjoyed can be frustrating.

Or even worse, forgetting how much you detested a recipe, just to prepare it once more and put up with it.

By continuously keeping a log of your favorite and least favorite dishes, you can avoid these culinary pitfalls.

Keeping track of any modifications you've made or would like to make to a specific recipe is especially useful if you want to fast advance from novice to master chef.

12. Always bring a list with you to the grocery store (or shop online).

Without a list, going to the grocery store will likely result in you spending a lot of time and money on unnecessary items.

Making a list can help you remain on task and resist the urge to buy food that you don't intend to eat just because it's on sale.

With regard to the area you live, several bigger grocery stores provide you the choice to shop online and have your groceries shipped or personally picked up at a specific time.

Although there may be a fee associated with using these services, they can be a terrific way to save time and stay away from the lengthy lineups and distracting store promotions.

13. Do not shop when you are hungry.

Avoid going to the grocery store when you're hungry since you're more prone to make impulsive purchases that you'll later regret.

Even though it differs from your usual meal and snack schedule, don't be afraid to eat a snack if you get the tiniest hint of hunger before you go shopping.

14. Purchase in large quantities

Utilize the bulk aisle at your neighborhood grocery stores to save funds, buy only what you require, and lessen wasteful packaging.

An excellent area to buy pantry essentials like rice, cereal, quinoa, almonds, seeds, dried fruit, and beans is in this section of the supermarket.

Provide your own packaging to avoid using disposable bags to transport your large purchases home.

15. Prepare for and utilize leftovers.

Plan to create enough food so there will be leftovers if you don't want to spend time cooking every day of the week.

Preparing a few more meals of whatever you're eating for dinner is a fantastic, effortless way to prepare for the following day's lunch.

If you are unhappy with left overs, consider how you might use them in another way so that they won't taste like leftovers.

For instance, if you roast a whole chicken with root vegetables for supper, you may use the leftover chicken by shredding it and adding it to tacos, soup, or salad the next day for lunch.

16. Group mix

Whenever you prepare a variety of meals in large quantities with the intention of using them in various ways during the week, you are cooking in groups. If you don't have much time to spend cooking during the week, this strategy is extremely helpful.

Consider preparing a sizable amount of quinoa or rice at the beginning of the week and roasting a large tray of vegetables, tofu, or meat to use in salads, stir-fries, scrambles, or grain bowls.

A bunch of chicken, tuna, or chickpea salad might also be prepared to be used in salads, on crackers, or in sandwiches.

17. Utilize your freezer.

You may save time, cut down on waste, and extend your food budget by cooking particular dishes or meals in bulk and freezing them for later use.

This technique may be applied to basic ingredients like broth, fresh bread, and tomato sauce as well as to complete meals like lasagna, soup, enchiladas, and breakfast burritos.

18. Prepare meals in advance.

A great meal prep technique is to pre-portion your meals into individual containers, especially if you're trying to consume a certain amount of food.

Professional athletes and workout fanatics who closely monitor their caloric intake and nutritional consumption frequently use this technique. When you're short on time, it's also a terrific way to promote weight loss or simply get ahead.

Make preparations for a substantial dinner with a minimum of 4-8 servings to benefit from this technique. Place each dish into a separate container and keep them chilled or frozen. Simply reheat and serve when ready.

19. Immediately wash and prepare fruits and vegetables.

Try cleaning and preparing fresh fruits and vegetables as soon as you arrive home from the farmer's market or the supermarket if your objective is to eat more of them.

You're more inclined to grab for those foods when you're feeling hungry if you open your pantry or freezer to discover a freshly made fruit smoothie or sticks of carrots and celery ready for nibbling.

It is simpler to resist eating a bag of potato chips or a plate of cookies just because they are quick and easy if you anticipate your hunger and prepare yourself with convenient and healthy options.

20. Prepare intelligently rather than laboriously

Don't be afraid to admit when you need to save money.

There are probably some healthy prepared options in your neighbourhood grocery shop if you don't have time to batch cook and portion your meals or aren't adept at chopping vegetables.

Pre-cut fruits and vegetables and prepared meals are typically more expensive, but if they help you eat more vegetables or reduce stress in your life, they could be well worth the extra cost.

Keep in mind that not everyone's meal preparation and planning procedures are the same. Long-term goal-sticking can be made easier if you have the wisdom to recognise when you need to cut back and increase efficiency.

21. Use a pressure or slow cooker.

When preparing meals, slow and pressure cookers can come in quite handy, especially if you don't have the time to stand at the stove.

With the help of these gadgets, cooking may be done more autonomously, allowing you to prepare meals while also performing other tasks or running errands.

22. Change the menu.

It's simple to fall into a diet rut and eat the same things every day.

Your meals may, at best, soon grow monotonous and cause you to lose your creative spark for cooking. The absence of variation may, at worst, result in nutrient deficits (4Trusted Source).

Make it a point to experiment with preparing different foods or meals on a regular basis to prevent this.

If you consistently select brown rice, consider switching to quinoa or barley. If you regularly eat broccoli, try switching it up with some cauliflower, asparagus, or romanesco.

You might also think about letting the changing of the seasons alter your menu. Consuming seasonal produce allows you to change up your diet while also saving money.

23. Make it pleasurable

If you enjoy doing it, you're more likely to maintain your new meal planning practise. Try to reframe it in your mind as a kind of self-care rather than something you must do.

If you're the cook at home, think about involving the whole family in meal preparation. In order to turn chopping vegetables or batch cooking soup into meaningful family time rather than simply another task, enlist the assistance of your family.

Put on your favourite music, a podcast, or an audiobook as you prepare meals alone if that's what you choose to do. It might soon become something you anticipate.

The end result
Making better food selections and saving time and money can both be accomplished via meal planning and preparation.

To lower your chance of acquiring conditions like high blood pressure, diabetes, and heart disease, eat a variety of foods from each food group.

Pick foods with low to no sodium, saturated fats, or added sugar.Try using fish, dairy, or fortified soy products along with beans, peas, and lentils in your meals to ensure that you consume adequate protein throughout the day and retain muscle mass.

Study up on protein and other essential vitamins and minerals.

Fruits and veggies can be cut or chopped and added to a variety of snacks and meals. When you have trouble slicing and chopping, look for pre-cut kinds. Try eating B12-fortified foods, like some cereals, or consult your physician about taking a vitamin B12 dietary supplement. Find out more about important minerals and vitamins.

By enhancing meals with plants and citrus, like lemon juice, you can reduce your salt intake. To stay hydrated and to promote nutrient absorption and meal digestion, drink plenty of water throughout the day. AVOID sugary beverages.

Although it might seem difficult at first, you can use these techniques to create a sustainable meal-planning routine that fits your particular lifestyle.

Creating a Balanced Diet plan for 30 days

Fruits, veggies, whole grains, dairy products, proteins, and beneficial oils are all part of a well-rounded eating plan. You can improve your insulin levels, lose weight, gain muscle, and other health and fitness objectives with the aid of a balanced eating plan.

You must take into account your calorie requirements, nutritional requirements, dietary choices, and lifestyle while developing a balanced diet plan for 30 days. To establish a diet plan that is balanced, you can use the following steps:

- Step 1: Establish your daily calorie requirements. Age, gender, height, weight, degree of activity, and health objectives all affect how many calories you need. An estimation of the number of calories required to maintain, lose, or gain weight can be made using a calorie counter.

- Step 2: Ascertain your dietary requirements. Your calorie requirements and health objectives will determine how much nutrition you require. A nutrition calculator can help you determine your daily requirements for protein, carbohydrates, fat, fiber, vitamins, and minerals. For basic advice on the kinds and serving sizes of foods you should eat, consult the Canada's Food Guide.

- Step 3: Look for recipes and meal suggestions that fit your interests and way of life. You can make a customised meal plan using a meal planner or a meal generator based on your dietary needs, spending limit, and schedule. Additionally, you can look through a number of cooking manuals or online resources that include nutritious dietary recommendations and recipes for a variety of cuisines.

- Step 4: Select your grocery items and write down your dietary plan. A documented meal plan can keep you on track and stop you from making rash selections. You can use a paper calendar, a computer programme, or an ordinary note on your refrigerator or phone. List every meal, snack, and beverage you intend to consume over the course of the following 30 days. Then list all the ingredients you need to buy on a shopping list. By doing this, you can avoid purchasing needless or unhealthy foods at the grocery shop and save both time and money.

- Step 5: Get your supplies ready and get cooking. Cooking over the week can be made simpler and quicker by prepping some or all of your supplies in advance. Vegetables can be chopped, grains or beans can be cooked, meats can be marinated, sauces or dressings can be made, and whole meals can even be assembled and stored in your containers until you're ready to consume them. You can also prepare food in large quantities and freeze some of it for later.

- Step 6: Assess and acknowledge your successes. Review your meal plan's effectiveness for yourself at the conclusion of the 30 days. Did you find the dishes tasty? Have you followed the plan? Have you achieved your goals? Which obstacles did you encounter? What can you change for the following time?

List of 30 meals to consider

Listed below is an exhaustive compilation of 30 meals you might want to add to your list of meals to plan. I will save the **recipes for these 30 meals for volume 2** of this book, which should be anticipated for, by mid October 2023.

1. Lemon-flavored chicken with rice

2. Cheese-topped Chipotle Mac

3. Broccoli and Chicken Casserole

4. Squash and corn soup

5. Southwest Flank Steak topped with Fresh Tomatillo Salsa

6.   Spinach,   feta,   and tzatziki-topped   Greek   turkey burgers

7. Stuffed spaghetti squash with cheese and spinach

8. Corn and rocket pizza with prosciutto

9. Fried "rice" made of cauliflower with chicken

10. Cobb Salad with Herb-Rubbed Chicken

11. Salmon in a Superfood Chopped Salad with Creamy Garlic Dressing

12.   Sausage   and   ricotta-topped macaroni

13. Chicken Verde Enchiladas

14. Sandwiches with quick pickles and slow-cooked brisket

15. Bowls of Asian Beef Noodles

16. Shrimp & Avocado Pesto over Zucchini Noodles

17. Spicy Stetson Chopped Salad

18. Avocados filled with salmon

19. Mini meatloaves with potatoes, green beans, and onions

20. White creamy chili with cream cheese

21. Speedy Puttanesca with prawns

22. Chickpea Curry

23.	Fried salmon with smoked chickpeas and greens

24. Lemon and Parmesan-Rubbed Chicken and Spinach Skillet Pasta

25.	Chicken-Cheddar-Broccoli Chowder

26. Flaky Fish Tacos that are Baked.

27. Potato and Curry Soup with Roasted Cauliflower

28. Lasagna with zucchini

29. Garlicky broccoli and pork chops

30. Slow-Cooker Chickpea and Chicken Soup with Mediterranean Flavors

It can be enjoyable and satisfying to make your food more tasty and fascinating. You may prepare excellent meals that will delight your palate and your health by utilizing a variety of cooking methods, ingredients, condiments, and recipes. I found the following advice on the internet:

- To brown your meat, poultry, or fish and add a deep flavor, use high-heat cooking techniques like pan-searing, grilling, broiling, or roasting. Simply take care not to overcook or burn your food as this might destroy the flavor and nutrients.

- Cook your vegetables slowly over low heat in a little oil, turning them occasionally, until they get brown and delicious. They can be used to prepare soups, sauces, or dish toppers for your main courses.

- When cooking meat or poultry, use the browned bits that stick to the bottom of the pan to make fond, which can be used to make a tasty sauce or gravy. Deglazing the pan involves adding liquid, such as wine, broth, or juice, and scraping out the browned parts with a wooden spoon.

- To improve the flavor of your food, use condiments of high quality. There are other alternatives available, including spicy pepper sauce, horseradish, wasabi, bean puree, flavored mustard, salsa, chutney, and wasabi.

- To give your meat, poultry, or fish more flavor and tenderness before cooking, marinate them. You can create your own marinade by combining oil, an acid (such vinegar or citrus juice), and additional seasonings.

- Add some acidic flavor by using lemon, lime, or orange zest (the grated peel) or citrus juice. Citrus fruits can add vitamin C2 and enhance and balance the flavor of your diet.

Take advantage of components with strong flavors sparingly, such as the seeds of pomegranates, chipotle pepper, cilantro, ginger, garlic, or mint. Without adding excessive calories, these ingredients can give your dishes a blast of flavor and color.

Additionally, you can attempt new dishes that suit your interests and way of life and get inspired by appropriate cookbooks, cookery programmes, and blogs. Try a variety of foods and eating regimens that offer a range of flavors and nutrients.

The Importance of Nutritious Rich Foods

Foods that are high in nutrients are those that are high in vitamins, minerals, and other health-promoting ingredients yet low in calories, sugar, sodium, and bad fats. Consuming foods high in nutrients can aid in the management or prevention of chronic illnesses like cancer, diabetes, and heart disease. Additionally, it can improve your immunity, assist your development and advancement, and help you keep a healthy weight.

Foods that are nutrient-rich include the following:

- Fruits and vegetables are abundant in fibre, antioxidants, vitamins C and A, potassium, and folate. They can aid in reducing inflammation, cholesterol, and blood pressure. Additionally, they can help your immune system and shield your cells from harm. Aim to consume 2.5 cups of veggies and 2 cups of fruit each day.

- Whole grains: These foods are high in selenium, iron, magnesium, fibre, and B vitamins. They can decrease your cholesterol, control your blood sugar, and prevent constipation. They can also boost your metabolism and provide you energy. At least 3 ounces of whole grains should be consumed each day.

- Lean protein: These foods are abundant in iron, zinc, vitamin B12, and protein. They can support the growth and repair of your blood, bones, skin, and muscles. Your immune system and hormone synthesis may also be supported by them. Aim to consume 5.5 ounces or more of lean protein per day. Lean proteins include things like beans, fish, chicken, eggs, nuts, and seeds.

- Low-fat dairy: These meals are a good source of calcium, phosphate, vitamin D, and protein. They can lower your blood pressure, strengthen your bones and teeth, and guard against osteoporosis. Additionally, they can help your muscles and nerves work. At least three cups of low-fat dairy products should be consumed each day. Dairy products that are low in fat include milk, yoghurt, cheese, and fortified soy milk.

These foods are high in monounsaturated fats as well as polyunsaturated omega-3 fatty acids, vitamin E, and phytochemicals, which are all considered healthy fats. They can assist in reducing your risk of heart disease, inflammation, and cholesterol. They can also safeguard the health of your eyes and brain. At least 5 teaspoons of good fats per day should be your goal. Olive oil, avocados, almonds, seeds, fatty seafood, and olive oil are a few examples of good fats.

You can use the following advice to eat rich and nutritious foods:

Select a range of foods from all the food groups every day. Consume more plant-based rather than animal-based foods. Select natural alternatives over finished or refined foods. Opt for fresh or frozen foods over canned or dried foods. Choose from low-sodium or no-salt-added foods over high-sodium or salt-added foods. Take to water or unsweetened beverages over sugary drinks.

Benefits of Healthy Eating for Adults

- May lengthen your life
- Supports muscles and maintains healthy skin, teeth, and eyes
- Increases immunity
- Bolsters the bones
- Reduces the risk of type 2 diabetes, heart disease, and several types of cancer
- Enhances the function of the digestive system and promotes healthy pregnancy and nursing
- Helps one reach and keep a healthy weight

Benefits of Healthy Eating for Children

- Aids muscles and maintains healthy skin, teeth, and eyes
- Helps one reach and keep an appropriate bodyweight
- Bolsters the bones
- Aids in brain growth
- Promotes wholesome growth
- Increases immunity
- Enhances the digestive system's performance

CONCLUSION

You have now finished reading this book, and hopefully you have gained a lot of knowledge regarding safe and quick weight loss. You now know your body type, how your metabolism works, and how weight loss works scientifically. Additionally, you have established useful deadlines, a calendar that can be used, and a 30-day diet plan that is balanced. You are now aware of the value of nutrient-dense foods and the advantages of good eating for both adults and children.

It's time to savour the fruits of your labour and to congratulate your accomplishments. By dropping pounds rapidly and successfully, you have changed both your body and your life. By embracing a healthy lifestyle, you have enhanced your well-being, disposition, and sense of self.

But your path does not finish here. To keep the weight off and stop it from regaining, there is still more to learn and do. Because of this, I have prepared a unique gift for you: Quick Pounds Shed volume 2!

This volume will teach you how to:

Increase your metabolism to burn more calories even when you're at rest, incorporate exercise into your daily routine without getting bored or overextended, and stay away from typical hazards and errors that can undermine your attempts to lose weight.
- Handle cravings, emotional eating, and stress-related eating -

Remain inspired and motivated to continue working towards your final objective

plus a lot more!

Keep checking back because this volume will soon be available. Don't pass up this chance to accelerate your weight loss. You merit it.

I appreciate you taking the time to read this book, and I hope you found it as enjoyable as I found it while writing it. I wish you ultimate success in your efforts to lose weight and beyond!

To be continued!